The Stigma of Growing Old in America:

A Personal Perspective

Pat Estelle

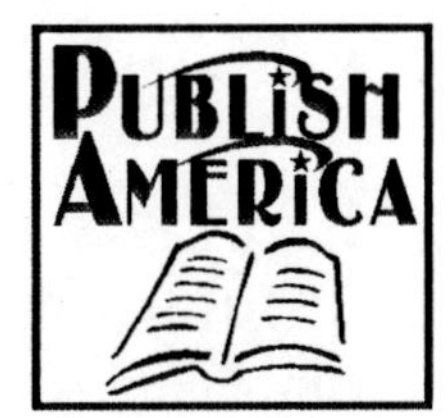

PublishAmerica

Baltimore

First printing

ISBN: 1-4137-4741-8
PUBLISHED BY PUBLISHAMERICA, LLLP
www.publishamerica.com
Baltimore

Printed in the United States of America

This book is dedicated to the loving memory of my mother.

A special thank-you to:
My friend, and a great librarian, Erlene Payne.
My niece, Charlene Sparks.
My brother, Jim Estelle & his wife, Dianne.

CHAPTER I – What *Old* Means.

As it relates to people, the word *old* cannot be easily defined, and is frequently used inappropriately if we accept the definitions provided by the Merriam-Webster dictionary: (1) the opposite of young (2) having lived or existed for a specified period of time (3) obsolete, and (4) no longer acceptable or useful.

Of course there is no argument that the first two can apply to people, but what about #3 and #4? There are millions who have reached the chronological age of seventy, eighty, or even greater, who are not obsolete, and are still quite useful and acceptable.

A thesaurus lists the most commonly used synonyms for old as: ancient, antique, time-worn, and antediluvian. It is my opinion that none of these accurately portray an "old" person, and could more appropriately be used to describe furniture, a used car, or vinyl records. "Mature in judgment" and "wise" are sometimes included as synonyms, and seem to be much more fitting, as are "perpetual" and "established."

Synonyms for the combined words, *"old-age,"* are: senescence, feebleness, weakness, infirmity, decrepitude, and dotage.

Those are especially difficult for me to accept, and I find *dotage* the most offensive. It's defined in the dictionary as: "a state or period of senile decay marked by decline of mental poise and alertness."

It seems obvious to me that when such words are ascribed to

human beings they evoke an image of a pathetic and pitiable creature. Then is it so surprising that such a representation of older people gives many a reason for embarrassment, shame, and even self-loathing?

But unless some miraculous scientific discovery has been made very recently, I'm afraid there is only one alternative to growing old, and that one is not particularly appealing to me at this time.

In my senior year of high school my chemistry teacher was only twenty-five years old, but much too old, I thought, to be flirting with the boys in my class. As an adolescent, an age difference of eight or nine years is seen much differently than such an age difference when you become a mature adult.

I probably resented the teacher's flirting only because she was so blatant in her favoritism, giving the boys better grades simply because she liked them more. It wasn't because the boys were smarter; forget the old gender-bias theory about boys being better in science and math.

At that age I placed older people into three categories: those who were past their teens, parents, then grandparents. But I don't recall thinking at any time that being old was some kind of detriment. Nor did it ever occur to me that there was discrimination or prejudice against anyone because of his or her age. Although I might have considered older people to have a flaw in judgment when it came to imposing their rules on others.

But that was a long time ago, and now that I presumably have reached my "golden years," (which I believe to begin at age sixty-five) I am sometimes confused as to how I should feel at this age. I don't believe it adheres to the persistent expectations of the majority.

I think a partial explanation for my confusion is that our society has, for inexplicable reasons, imposed on older people conditions and standards of conduct that appear to be completely arbitrary.

The rules seem to differ noticeably, depending on one's social and/or economic status. One's ideology, political persuasion, and religious beliefs also seem to affect the way in which they're treated by society; whether or not they're valued and respected. And since there is no actual rule book, I'm not always sure of what is or is not acceptable.

What is quite clear, however, to all of us older Americans, is that we're expected to act with dignity and decorum at all times. The slightest impropriety is totally unacceptable. Some of the tacit rules follow:

We should not be overly demonstrative in public. We're expected to sit quietly, smile, (but never laugh too loudly) and make every attempt not to cry or exhibit anger or frustration. If we can avoid exhibiting any of these emotions, perhaps we won't be labeled "that crazy old lady," or "poor old thing."

It's not considered dignified or proper to drive a sports car or a convertible. If you're driving around in a beautiful car with the top down, you'll likely hear some remark such as "he's in his second childhood," or "why in the world would an old lady buy a car like that!"

It might be best in the presence of some not to disclose your interests – if you still like Rock & Roll music that's a clear indication that you're a bit weird. You must be more subtle in your tastes, and that includes your music.

You must dress conservatively, and appropriately for your age; otherwise there will be various disapproving comments, such as, "she's just too old to be wearing that."

If a thief tells you to hand over your wallet or purse, you're expected to do as he says – never mind that you hold a 1st Degree Black Belt in Karate. After all, you're old and weak, and just too vulnerable.

Do not let it be known that you own a motorcycle, and that you actually *ride it*! First of all, that would be to contravene the rule of "act with dignity and decorum at all times." And you know that riding a motorcycle is too dangerous; old people shouldn't be taking such risks – you'll hurt yourself, or someone else.

Of course I'm just being facetious, but are you beginning to get the picture? There *is* a *stigma*; older people are in a clear and distinct state of disfavor.

When considering this unfavorable attitude directed toward older people, it comes as no surprise that many will lie about their age, or simply refuse to reveal it. Actually this practice begins long before we become senior citizens.

The "oldest-old" are probably less likely to deny their true age; perhaps they even brag about it. Denying your age when you reach ninety or one hundred years probably doesn't occur to you. After all, it should be considered a badge of honor.

Another real problem for me which doesn't seem to be directed only toward senior citizens, is when people make remarks such as, "she sure doesn't look her age," or "doesn't she look terrific for fifty-one," or "he can't possibly be sixty-five years old." That seems to support the idea that we're preoccupied with age.

An example of this occurred recently on a television program in which there was interaction with the audience; one lady said, "today's my birthday – I'm seventy years old."

That seemed to generate shock and dismay, and there were such exclamations as, "wow, are you really seventy – I would never believe that." Other expressions of disbelief could be heard, suggesting that maybe it wasn't actually true. After all, if you're "that old," how is it possible to look so great? But most remarks were made with sincere admiration, and the lady expressed her thanks for the compliments.

But isn't it reasonable to assume that if you're making

informed decisions about your health; i.e., eating properly, exercising, maintaining a healthy weight, and managing stress, that you will *look* and *feel* terrific? There are many, many senior citizens who are doing just that. They're educating themselves; learning more about proper nutrition, appropriate exercises, meditation and relaxation techniques. No doubt most are delighted with the results.

I would like to suggest that it's a much greater compliment simply to say to a person, "you look terrific," or "wow, you're really in great shape." In my judgment, the appended "for your age" is definitely not necessary.

CHAPTER II – Physical Changes.

Realistically, of course, we know that as we age there are physical changes that take place, and alter our appearance to some degree. Therefore, one can be certain that a person who has reached the age of sixty or sixty-five will never be mistaken for a twenty- or thirty-year-old, even if he or she is extremely healthy, and/or has had extensive cosmetic surgery.

Likewise, a person who is sixty years old, and made the decision to give up some bad habits, and modify his or her lifestyle at an earlier age, will not appear to be in such declining years as the sixty-year-old person whose lifestyle leaves much to be desired.

But who decided what a sixty-year-old should look like, or a seventy-year-old? Is it based on how people of that age might have appeared a hundred years ago? With the life expectancy of that period, there were very, very few who reached such an age. At the turn of the twentieth century, life expectancy in the United States was only forty-nine years.

Granted, at some time in our history, especially when people were not expected to live past the age of thirty or forty years, one might be able to make a pretty good guess as to one's age based on his or her appearance, at least within a couple of years. But the life expectancy in the United States at the end of the twentieth century was seventy-seven years!

Still we persist in thinking that our chronological age is the main determinant in what our physical "look" should be.

Of course it is generally easy to identify teens by their appearance; the age of young adults can also be approximated within perhaps a four or five year range. After that I think it is very difficult to "guess" a person's age.

An experiment that might prove how difficult it is to judge one's age is to place ten people who are between the ages of thirty and forty, or those between fifty and sixty, in a room together. In my experience, it has been practically impossible to guess anyone's age. It is only possible to come within six or eight years of the actual age of a few.

So I think it's important to remember that the physical appearance is not necessarily an indicator of one's chronological age. Also, the chronological age is not a measure of *dotage*. Don't you agree that word is repugnant?

I think we can assume that studies have been conducted in an attempt to determine the amount of damage and deterioration that takes place within cells in any given time, thereby reducing the function of bodily organs.

But the way in which people age can vary dramatically; the degree of damage to cells may be very different. Lifestyle, environmental, and genetic factors are, in part, responsible for the marked variations of how well people can function, physically or mentally, at any given age.

Furthermore, if we're in good physical and mental health, and all the internal organs are functioning as they should, is the exterior really that important? It is my opinion that when a person can meet those exacting standards, there should be no fear of dotage, even if one has reached what is commonly referred to as elderly.

But there is no denying that most of us really do *feel* better if we think we *look* pretty good. And I'm of the opinion that we should definitely try to look our best at all times.

It's no secret that the mind and body work conjointly. All of our thoughts, our emotions, all mental activity cause various chemicals or substances to be released from our brain, which can have an effect on our body.

So if our emotional state is good, if we are confident and self-assured, that means we will be healthier, and also look better. "Don't Worry, Be Happy," a song written and sung by Bobby McFerrin a few years ago, sounds like very good advice for anyone, but is not so easy to follow.

Actually it rarely occurs to me that I'm now considered to be "old." However, I only need to look at my face in a mirror, and it becomes clear that I am no longer young. It is apparent that I look different than when I was twenty-five or thirty years old. But that "look" reflects who I am, my history; a life filled with happiness, sadness, joy, pain, love, and heartbreak. And it won't deter me from being all that I can be, and doing everything that I want to do. I place few limitations on myself; if I feel I'm physically and/or mentally capable of undertaking a new task, project, or adventure, I will totally ignore the admonition of "you're too old."

I assume our government is responsible for affixing the traditional "old age" at sixty-five years. It was probably an arbitrary number based on the fact that sixty-five was the age at which we were expected to retire; from our jobs, that is.

But it's clear to me that there are significant differences between a sixty-five-year-old at the time I was an adolescent, and those in the present day; one of the most important being that we aren't sitting around in our rocking chairs, waiting to die.

At first glance, when I'm fully clothed, I appear to be much the same as I did forty-five years ago, but there are obvious physical changes. Thankfully, my weight remains the same, within six or eight pounds; and my height is the same; I didn't shrink even one inch.

But that certainly doesn't mean my body actually looks the same as when I was twenty years old; nothing is tight, firm, or smooth. There is loose skin, thin skin, brown spots, and other little wart-like growths, which the doctor informs me are called seborrheic keratoses. I'm told they are quite common in older people and are completely harmless. And of course they can be removed cryogenically.

There is hair now growing on parts of my body where it never grew before, and significant loss of hair in areas where it was once abundant. One disturbing example which immediately comes to mind is that I now have so few eyelashes that they can hardly be seen; long, lush eyelashes are definitely a thing of the past. And even though false eyelashes might be a viable solution for some, I have not opted for those.

I can no longer see how to read without glasses, which is a common vision problem that affects many people by the age of forty, and almost everyone eventually. I've learned that this condition is known as Presbyopia, and occurs as the lens becomes less flexible and loses its ability to focus. As a result, one's vision becomes blurred when trying to read or focus on close-up objects.

Until recently the only solution was to wear glasses, but in March of 2004, the FDA approved a procedure called NearVision CK (Conductive Keratoplasty), which is apparently minimally invasive and safe for people over the age of forty who have had good vision their entire life and now require reading glasses.

Since I don't require them for distance, I'm continuously taking the glasses off and putting them on again, which is a nuisance. The new technology sounds like a wonderful way to solve that problem.

Another disturbing change began to occur at about the age of fifty-five; and that was in my customary sleep patterns, how much and how well I slept, etc. That was probably the most unsettling change, except for the post-menopausal difficulties that I experienced, and thankfully those were eventually resolved with hormone treatment.

It is my understanding that many women go through menopause with very few problems. Unfortunately I was not one of them. Until I chose hormone replacement therapy as the solution, I endured unrelenting "hot flashes" and "night sweats."

The medical profession has informed us that hormone replacement therapy may increase the risk of heart attacks and strokes. But if I were still experiencing those serious menopausal symptoms, I would not hesitate to resume hormone treatment. It is my belief that the benefits far outweigh the small risk involved, and it is not an exaggeration to say that I survived the years after menopause only because of HRT. There are probably millions of women who share that sentiment.

However, I do feel fortunate at this time that there are only three significant changes I find somewhat troublesome: (1) the body hair situation; (2) the necessity for reading glasses; and (3) the alteration in my sleep patterns.

And since there is now a possible permanent solution for the vision problem, I may only have to deal with two minor maladies. I think the hair definitely will continue to come and go – nothing I can do about that. And I've already adjusted pretty well to the disruption in my sleeping habits.

But I do think it would be wonderful to sleep eight or nine consecutive hours, without interruption, regardless of the time I go to bed – I long for those days.

However, since I do sleep about seven hours each night, and am told that's exactly what I need, there's actually no reason for concern. My predicament is certainly not insomnia; there's no sleep deprivation.

Over a period of time I've made minor adjustments which relieved some of my early anxiety.

Even though I'm not always successful, I try for a regular bedtime; listen to soft music or relaxation tapes when it takes more time to fall asleep; and I no longer panic when I suddenly awake for no apparent reason.

The minor revisions and modifications that are now required cause little apprehension, and hopefully I will never have first-hand knowledge of anything more vexing.

It is important, however, that I make this point: I'm so very, very thankful that these physical and physiological changes occur gradually over a period of years. If this happened overnight, or even over the period of *one* year, it would be such a shock, such a traumatic event, that some of us might choose that "alternative" to which I alluded earlier.

We know, of course, that there are various means available for improving our physical appearance. It is possible to eliminate the wrinkles, the loose, sagging skin, and the stretch marks, etc.

There is collagen or other substances that can be injected into any or all parts of the body to smooth out or plump-up where needed, and fat can be extracted from any or all parts, and the excess skin can be removed.

Of course there's the traditional face-lift, the brow-lift, and the tummy-tuck. There are hair transplants; there's botox; there is laser whitening to make our teeth beautiful; anything that is needed for a complete "make-over."

I think cosmetic surgery can be very useful; I wouldn't hesitate to take advantage of the skill and expertise of a qualified and experienced surgeon if I were in a financial position to do so. But if I'm realistic when attempting to calculate the sum required to meet my goals, I acknowledge that the cost would be prohibitive, and I quickly dismiss the idea.

Even though it is my opinion that cosmetic surgery is not often undertaken for the purpose of actually denying one's age, or refusing to accept his or her own mortality, there are instances of it being used for the wrong reasons. But I hope most of us are mature enough to recognize that "looking good" doesn't necessarily make us well-adjusted and happy.

I believe, though, cosmetic surgery can help some people to validate their own worth and usefulness in a society that criticizes and denounces those who are no longer physically attractive.

And we know that the metamorphosis generally accompanying the ageing process is not considered to be attractive.

But the harsh reality is that most older Americans are not in a financial position to afford such luxuries as cosmetic surgery. As a matter of fact, many are living in poverty. Their priorities are food, shelter, clothing, and medical care.

The Federal Administration on Ageing indicates that in the year 2001, there were 3.4 million senior citizens living below the poverty level. This means an annual income of $9,000 for one individual, or $12,000 for a couple. An additional 2.2 million seniors were considered to be "near poor."

And according to U.S. Statistics, there were an estimated 35 million Americans over the age of sixty-five living in the United States in the year 2000.

When considering the problems and difficulties with which many senior citizens are faced daily, the concerns about wrinkles or similar matters are of no consequence, and seem trivial and unimportant.

Furthermore, no amount of plastic surgery will make you healthy; yes, temporary improvement in your emotional state no doubt; which, in turn, will have an overall positive effect. But our primary focus should be about taking better care of ourselves, doing what we know will improve our quality of life.

But as with any other segment of society, senior citizens are a diverse group, and their needs and wishes vary. Even as we remain cognizant of the shameful conditions that plague many, we are often self-absorbed, with neither the time nor the inclination to worry about those who are less fortunate. Admittedly, a certain degree of selfishness is probably inherent in all of us.

I do believe, however, that it is important not to engage in feelings of guilt, or to deny ourselves those things we can and should do that will improve our own life, and significantly impact our future good health and happiness. Obviously more options are available to those who are financially solvent.

In spite of all the vicissitudes of time, I consider myself to be relatively happy and contented, with an even temperament and a positive outlook on life. I am in excellent health, and wish everyone could be so fortunate. I have many interests, but am always eager to learn and experience new things.

And even though I think I'm dealing with the transition into old age in the best possible way, I'm still baffled by it all. I don't understand why just the word "old" can conjure up negative images, and that misconceptions and stereotypes are reinforced by the general attitude of our society.

No one wants to grow old. I don't recall ever having heard a person say, "Oh, I'll sure be happy when I get old." We're more likely to hear the kind of comments that warn us of the "dangers" that lie ahead. Is it possible that a fear of becoming unattractive, and enduring pain and suffering, are responsible for the prevailing attitude? Or is it simply our fear of death? Only very young children want to be older, and of course teenagers are anxious to reach the age of twenty-one.

I recall an incident from many years ago on the twenty-eighth birthday of my older sister. Everyone was having cake and ice cream, celebrating the occasion, when suddenly my sister began crying and exclaimed, "Oh, I'm getting so old – just look at me!"

There were smiles and reassurances from others, but it was not a funny situation; my sister was obviously distraught. In retrospect, the incident seems a bit silly, but it was a serious matter to her at the time.

And more recently, on the twenty-fifth birthday of my godson, he expressed a similar viewpoint. When someone asked him how it felt to be twenty-five years old, he said, "I feel like I'm really getting on up there – twenty-five is pretty old."

That seems to be the sentiment of many that age – they believe their strengths, abilities, and prowess are already beginning to ebb.

It is my opinion that we place far too much emphasis on our age and our looks. But there is empirical evidence to show that people who are regarded as "beautiful" or "pretty" receive preferential treatment.

And since the general consensus is that we "lose" our looks as we age, the correlation between the two seems clear.

But how did we ever reach this point? Were the early humans concerned about their appearance? Maybe not! They were probably far too busy just trying to survive.

Of course we know the story of Narcissus in Greek mythology. After seeing his beautiful reflection in a pool, he fell in love with himself, then just pined away, died, and was changed into a flower. I think there are other versions of what happened to him, but I like the idea that he was changed into a flower.

It seems that for thousands of years people have gone to great lengths to make themselves attractive or beautiful.

Ancient civilizations, particularly Egypt, were very concerned about beauty and body care; cleanliness, personal hygiene, preventing odors, etc. (And I applaud all those, here and now, who are eager to prevent odors and have an interest in personal hygiene).

Preserved artifacts from excavations have revealed cosmetic implements, even a kind of tweezers. Wig boxes, and containers of various creams, unguents and oils were discovered. There was also Kohl, which was a kind of preparation to darken the eyelids.

Egypt's queen Cleopatra is credited with writing a book of beauty secrets around 50 B.C. And of course about 1300 years earlier, there was Egypt's most famous queen, Nefertiti, who is known for her beauty.

I've also read about an ancient Egyptian manuscript entitled, *The Beginning of the Book on How to make the Old Young*. You can bet that would be on the Bestsellers' list in the United States, and probably elsewhere.

At least since Biblical times people have thought the black mud from the Dead Sea, which contains natural salt and minerals, has therapeutic qualities, and helps to stimulate and revitalize the skin.

Apparently the interest in these beauty and body-care products transcended gender lines; men also used them. And things really haven't changed in that regard.

Most of us primp and preen now and then, and spend a lot of time grooming and adorning ourselves with baubles or jewels. We make an effort to look our very best, especially when we're trying to impress others, most often the opposite sex.

But beauty is only a concept, which differs greatly from culture to culture. And *inner beauty* is much more important, even though such a statement sounds clichéd and trite.

Here's an interesting quote about beauty from the eighteenth century philosopher and historian, David Hume: "Beauty is no quality in things themselves. It exists merely in the mind which contemplates them; and each mind perceives a different beauty."

And from the well-known film star, Jacqueline Bisset: "Character contributes to beauty – a mode of conduct, a standard of courage, discipline, fortitude, and integrity can do a great deal to make a woman beautiful."

But perhaps this quotation from Shakespeare says it best, at least for women: ""Tis beauty that doth oft make women proud; 'tis virtue that doth make them most admired; 'tis modesty that makes them seem divine."

One advantage of not being blessed with beauty is that the physical effects of ageing are far less likely to cause us serious anxiety or grief.

CHAPTER III – Discrimination and Maltreatment.

A very real concern for all of us should be about the mistreatment, the abuse, the discrimination against senior citizens, and the general attitude of society. Here are just a few examples about which I've read, experienced personally, or heard from acquaintances:

Most of us know someone who has been pressured to retire from his or her job because of their age, in spite of the Federal Age Discrimination in Employment Act, (ADEA) which is supposed to protect workers over the age of forty.

In an Associated Press article which I read on the Internet in April, 2004, a sixty-two-year-old woman filed a lawsuit against Domino's Pizza for age discrimination. She apparently worked there for twenty years, and claims that she was fired and replaced with a younger worker.

Another article tells of a woman in her mid-fifties who had worked for the Girl Scouts for more than twenty-one years, and alleges that she was dismissed and replaced by a younger employee. She also alleged that an executive director said she wanted "young, beautiful" people to work there. The former employee filed a lawsuit and won.

I know of an individual who was told a few years ago when computers were becoming more common in the workplace that she was "too old" to learn how to operate a computer, and that perhaps she might want to consider other employment.

And like so many of us, she didn't want the hassle of dealing with a team of company lawyers. It wouldn't be easy in the best of circumstances to prove discrimination, but for one lone employee it would be almost impossible. The charge would have to be more than just a few words spoken by her employer, regardless of how odious.

She felt that it was a no-win situation; requiring time, energy, and money which she was not prepared to expend. Also, she would need a thick skin, and be able to handle stress well. So she forfeited even before the fight began.

I'm happy to report that when I last heard, she had another job and was quite happy. But "all's well that ends well" is not necessarily a satisfactory conclusion.

There are other instances of older people applying for a job, and being bluntly told by the employer in the interview that they are looking for a younger person. The Federal Age Discrimination in Employment Act is simply ignored.

That's a clear indication that there is a bias, and even though the older person may very well be more qualified and have more experience, the employer doesn't acknowledge that he or she could be an asset.

To give employers the benefit of the doubt, I suppose that hiring a younger person is sometimes done for financial reasons. The employer can probably pay a lesser salary to the younger individual. But in many instances, the reason for not hiring the applicant is because he or she is considered to be too old.

And who are the first employees to go when a company decides to "down-size?" The older workers, of course. And it's not easy to prove differently when the employer explains that the reason for the dismissal is strictly financial – gotta consider that bottom line!

I once read about a physician who was not allowed to work at a particular medical facility when he reached the age of seventy, even though he was in excellent health. He was simply told by the "powers that be" that he was too old to treat patients.

Not very long ago, while having dinner in a restaurant, I overheard a part of the conversation between two women, and seriously began to eavesdrop when one of them said her boss had jokingly told her that perhaps if she had a face-lift she could "keep up" with the younger employees. I was unable to hear the remainder of the conversation, but if her boss actually said that, it probably wasn't in jest. What a great joke; to think that the company might increase production by encouraging older employees to have a face-lift! I'm sure most people would not find that amusing.

Other ways in which older citizens are treated differently is in the insurance industry. Some companies simply will not insure a person of a certain age.

There are also instances where specified coverage is limited or totally excluded; mental health treatment is an example where some insurers will not cover a person after the age of sixty-five, at least that was the practice of some insurance companies in the past.

And the Equal Employment Opportunity Commission (EEOC) in April of 2004 voted to allow employers to reduce or eliminate health benefits for retirees when they become eligible for Medicare at age sixty-five. The EEOC claims that such cuts do not violate the civil-rights law banning age discrimination.

I say that they're wrong – it definitely is age discrimination! And there are probably millions of Medicare recipients who would agree. Many are receiving health benefits from their former employers, and are presumably distressed and anxious about that decision.

But the maltreatment and discrimination of older people is rampant, and certainly not limited to insurance companies and other places of employment.

A very real and common type of discrimination occurs in some of the car rental agencies. They set an age limit for those renting cars, even when the person requesting the car has a valid drivers' license and a good driving record.

There is also age discrimination in the television, movie and music industries. It was reported in the national news in March, 2004, that Dick Clark's production company was being sued for age discrimination by a seventy-six-year-old game show producer, whom Clark had allegedly refused to hire.

The article listed Dick Clark's age as seventy-four. It went on to say that sometime in the year 2003 the man seeking employment received a personal letter from Dick Clark. He allegedly explained his reasons for denying the man a job, saying, "people our age are considered dinosaurs, the business is being run by the next generation." The game show producer claimed to have been "embarrassed," "humiliated," and "aggravated."

I am not a big TV fan, but have observed enough to know that the few senior citizens I've seen are not usually presented in a positive role. They're often portrayed as the "grouchy old man," "the bitchy old lady," or someone silly and forgetful, approaching senility.

As for TV advertising, the only seniors I see in commercials are extolling the miracles of medicine. They tout the cures for arthritis, osteoporosis, high cholesterol, deep vein thrombosis, and constipation. And a few can be seen suggesting all kinds of help for denture wearers. Occasionally, with tricks of the camera, something outrageous and unrealistic like an eighty-five-year-old lady doing back flips or pole-vaulting, can be seen. Of course she can do that because she drinks some kind of juice.

Only younger people seem to buy cars, appliances, or furniture. They also seem to be the only ones using cosmetics and hair products, or drinking beer. There is one exception I noticed in the cosmetic industry ads. A beautiful woman with a flawless complexion, and not even the tiniest line or wrinkle on her face, and claiming to be in the "over fifty" crowd, advertises a face cream or moisturizer. Using that product is the reason she has no wrinkles. Yeah, right!

Sometimes there is discrimination against older people when trying to find suitable housing – especially in some rental areas. They're given various reasons for denial of their rental application, but frequently are thought to be "unacceptable" as tenants simply because they're too old.

There are many rental and/or condominium complexes that are designated specifically for senior citizens. Whether or not a person wishes to live in such a location should be a personal choice, and not obligatory.

For many years I've been donating blood to the blood bank of the city in which I live. My blood is extremely valuable to them since I am what is known as a "universal donor." The blood bank does not hesitate to call and ask me to donate every eight weeks, the period of time required between donations.

But I have been informed that I can no longer donate when I reach the age of sixty-nine years. I once asked the reason for that, and the person to whom I directed the question was unable to give me a satisfactory answer. So I'm left once again to think that it's simply another example of discrimination.

Perhaps I should consult a doctor, or do some extensive research to determine why my blood ceases to be of any value at the age of sixty-nine. I acknowledge that a "cut-off" date may sometimes be necessary, but if a person is in good health, with no medical problems, isn't imposing such an age limit inappropriate and unfair? Oh well, that will be the blood bank's loss, not mine!

Many seniors do not receive quality health care, which of course is a kind of discrimination, or perhaps just neglect. Their ailments are often ignored, and there is sometimes the suggestion that nothing is wrong, that "it's all in your head," when they attempt to explain their symptoms to a doctor.

Time and again, because of pre-conceived notions, complaints that are thought to be age-related are not taken seriously, and there is little effort made to get to the core of the problem. And much too frequently, in my view, the physician prescribes more medication that is not really needed. He or she appears to be indifferent to the needs of the patient.

An incident that occurred with an acquaintance of mine a few years ago underscores the necessity for more geriatric training in the medical field. The woman was about sixty-two years old at the time. While consulting her physician for some other condition, she also asked for advice on how to treat extremely dry skin. The doctor simply told her to bathe less frequently. I didn't bother to ask if she complied.

Of course her problem could easily have been resolved without the assistance of a physician. However, there are those who choose not to make use of their own common sense abilities. Still, I consider the advice of her doctor to be ludicrous – downright absurd!

If a doctor is unable to make a diagnosis, or cannot offer an acceptable answer or solution for a problem, the patient should be referred to someone who can.

Regardless of age, each person is entitled to the best possible medical care. And even though the patient should understand and accept his share of responsibility regarding health issues, there can sometimes be plausible explanations which make that impossible.

There can be problems of communication between the doctor and patient because of language, or lack of education. And there are some people who have an unnatural trust in their doctor; a blind loyalty that prevents them from questioning the physician's advice or instructions.

Doctors are not infallible; patients *should* ask questions. It's important to know when given the doctor's diagnosis exactly what it means, and the prognosis of the disease or illness, what can be anticipated. I like to know what results are to be achieved from the prescribed medication; possible side effects, drug interactions, etc.

According to statistics on the Internet from the National Academy on an Ageing Society, and Alliance for Ageing Research, the sixty-five-plus group of Americans represent only 12% of the population, but use one-third of all health care services provided, and occupy one-half of all physician time.

I was dismayed to read that patients sixty-five years old and older visit doctors an average of 11.4 times a year. Patients who are at least eighty-five years of age visit a doctor an average of 15 times each year. Those between the ages of forty-five and sixty-five visit a doctor an average of 7.2 times yearly.

But that time spent pursuing medical attention doesn't necessarily translate into genuine concern, consideration, and dedication on the part of those providing the required services.

I believe it's possible to deliver better quality care to the elderly if more health professionals are trained in the field of geriatrics, and more attention is given to preventive and rehabilitative medicine. The old saying of "an ounce of prevention is worth a pound of cure," is true, and should be considered as sound advice. It is possible to actually stop an illness, to stop a disease, before it can happen.

The statistics from the sources mentioned above, indicate that only three of the country's 145 medical schools have a full-scale department of geriatrics that require mandatory rotation of students and residents. If this is accurate information, it means less than 3% of all medical students take even one course in geriatrics. It's clear there is a need for many more.

Therefore, I don't believe we can assume that all physicians are equipped to provide the best medical assistance for senior citizens.

We know that many injuries and illnesses, the overdosing and misuse of medications, even some hospitalizations, could be prevented if patients received more information and counseling. Instructions on the proper way to take their medication, the devastating effects of interaction with other drugs or alcohol, the importance of a proper diet, incorporating some kind of activity into their routine, are all important.

With more geriatric training, physicians might be able to prevent the onset of myriad disorders that are common among the elderly; provide ways to improve their hearing, and correct their vision. More information and suggestions for the treatment of arthritis could be offered. And if patients were more closely monitored for high blood pressure, and received proper treatment, the risk of strokes could be reduced.

There could, and should, be discussions between physician and patient about safety measures to take in their homes. Recommendations on how to improve balance, coordination, and mobility could drastically reduce the number of fall-related injuries suffered by senior citizens.

According to information from the Centers for Disease Control and Prevention (CDC), the cost for fall-related injuries in the year 2000 was estimated to be $20.2 billion. Now that's incredible!

Health-care workers who have had proper training are more

likely to monitor post-menopausal women for low bone mineral density (BMD). Osteoporosis is a serious problem, and with early treatment can often be prevented, or for those who are already affected by the disease, the damage can be partially reversed with medications that actually stimulate bone growth.

One of the devastating results of osteoporosis in post-menopausal women is compression fractures of the vertebrae, as well as other fractures. These women become frail and vulnerable; and often after numerous fractures, they're unable to resume their normal activities.

Even though osteoporosis is much more common among women, The National Osteoporosis Foundation estimates that approximately two million men in the United States have the disease, and possibly twelve million more are at risk. But apparently it remains underdiagnosed among men, and has not received adequate research.

There are also seniors who have vitamin and mineral deficiencies that might be suspected as the cause of some ailments presented by patients; these deficiencies could be easily detected, and effectively corrected. That might prevent more serious problems from occurring in the future. It's not possible for most of us to receive sufficient amounts of vitamins and minerals in the foods we consume, many of which are absolutely essential in maintaining good health.

Much more attention to these potentially disabling infirmities requires the efforts and dedication of adequately trained health care professionals, working with informed and knowledgeable patients.

Even though we are sometimes given conflicting information from the medical and scientific field of experts, we must be discerning, and aggressively attempt to make wise and intelligent decisions as to what will best ensure our own good health.

Health professionals play a very important role in advising, educating, and caring for the ill and afflicted, and I believe the majority are resolute and dedicated. But it is my opinion that too many physicians are excessive in prescribing pills that are not necessary. The results can be disastrous.

I have had personal experience with relatives who were prescribed far too much medication, most of which they did not need. It was often a simple matter of "ask, and you shall receive."

Also, I have known several people in the past who were addicted to prescription drugs, one of whom was addicted for many years, and has been rehabilitated. He now refers to himself as a "recovering addict" and told me how difficult it was for him.

A personal experience of what I perceived to be neglect and maltreatment on the part of health care workers occurred a couple of years ago. I was hospitalized for a few days when I had total knee replacement surgery, and my brief stay was unpleasant, to say the least.

More often than not a total knee replacement is performed on patients who are more than sixty years old – and of course my records would have revealed my age to the staff. It soon became clear to me that they had a fixed idea, an undesirable stereotype of an old person, believing that most of us are senile, or to some degree mentally impaired, that we can't hear, can't see, that we're incontinent, etc.

I was not physically abused by anyone, but on two occasions there were angry verbal attacks by a nurse. I won't attempt to explain what presumably provoked her, but the nurse's conduct was very unprofessional, and not warranted.

I had mistakenly assumed that concern, compassion, and understanding were inherent in professional health care workers. If not, why in the world, I wondered, would they undertake such demanding work? And to be fair, I'm certain there are many who are compassionate, caring, and understanding. However, I wasn't so fortunate as to encounter anyone possessing those qualities during my hospital stay.

My needs and requests were often ignored; there were absolutely inexcusable delays when I requested pain medication. When a nurse or an aide deigned to assist me, it was the action of an automaton, devoid of empathy or feeling.

As a vegetarian I had told my doctor and the hospital registration office in advance that my diet could not contain meat. After receiving my first meal with meat, I once again asked a registered nurse to please inform the kitchen of my special dietary needs. Then I received my second meal without the necessary changes, and it was clear they had made no effort to grant my request.

On the second day of my confinement, I asked a nurse for the telephone number of the kitchen where the patients' food was prepared. I called the kitchen and explained my situation, and was told they had not received a request from the nursing staff for a vegetarian meal. They did immediately solve the problem, and from that point forward I received food I could eat. My impression was that the nursing staff simply didn't want to be bothered, and that they made their own decision as to what should be included in their "job description."

My room was in close proximity to the nurses' station, and I could often hear what was being said by the staff. On more than one occasion I heard them discussing the patients, sometimes making a disparaging comment. One of the patients apparently was a very old man, and the staff would make a derisive and belittling remark about him, then really laugh about it.

I am well aware that the job of a nurse is not easy; there is often a shortage of staff and they're required to work overtime. The work is physically demanding, and there are difficult patients with whom they must deal each and every day.

And being cognizant of the fact that perhaps they were overworked, I tried hard to be agreeable and make no unnecessary demands, but that didn't protect me from their contempt.

After being released, I wrote an official letter of complaint to the hospital administration, with a copy to the surgeon, and expressed myself in very forceful terms. Perhaps more of us should write letters, make telephone calls, and do whatever is necessary to try and prevent that kind of treatment.

I received a letter of response from the hospital, assuring me that a copy of my letter would be forwarded to the Director of Nursing, and that steps would be taken to avoid similar occurrences in the future.

The administration of any facility where an act of mistreatment, discrimination, or abuse takes place should be made aware of it in the most emphatic way. That kind of conduct should not be tolerated.

In the past I spent some time as a volunteer in a nursing home. I observed numerous incidents of verbal abuse and neglect. There were many times when I heard patients saying, "please help me," sometimes actually screaming, and they would be ignored. An aide might actually pass by the patient's room and never even look inside.

As a volunteer, I was not allowed to actually perform any kind of personal care, but there were times when I would try to seek help for them. And on more than one occasion when I boldly informed a staff member that the individual needed attention, I was told he or she was a trouble-maker; there was nothing really wrong, and that ultimately you take little notice of the screaming and crying. I consider that to be an example of contempt and disdain for the patients.

Many of the patients were placed in wheelchairs, taken into the "day-room" after breakfast, and left completely unattended until lunch time. Some appeared to be heavily medicated, and unable to even hold up their head. Few showed any interest in the program appearing on the screen of the television set in the room. There were no other available forms of recreation or entertainment.

There was often urine on the floor under the wheelchairs – apparently there were no adult diapers available there! They were dejected, dispirited, forgotten, and lonely people, forced to live in abominable circumstances.

Since my experience as a volunteer, I have had occasion to visit other nursing facilities in three different states. I saw little or no difference in their operations, or in the service they provide. The maltreatment seems to be pervasive.

Once, while visiting my uncle in a nursing home, and during the course of a conversation with another visitor, I unabashedly expressed my view of such facilities, and how I thought it would be so depressing to live in such a wretched place. The lady smiled and said, "Well, you should get used to the idea, because if you live, you'll end up in one some day." What a disturbing possibility!

In a report prepared by the Special Investigations Division of the minority staff of the Government Reform Committee for U.S. Representative, Henry A. Waxman, in July 2001, there are shocking examples of physical, sexual, and verbal abuse of patients in the nursing homes of the United States.

The report states that in a two-year period from January 1, 1999 through January 1, 2001, there were 5,283 nursing homes cited for an abuse violation, all of which had the potential to harm residents. In over 1600 of those homes, the violations were serious enough to actually cause bodily harm, or placed the residents in immediate jeopardy of death or serious injury.

The report goes on to say that it is very likely the findings actually *underestimate* the incidence of abuse in nursing homes, that many go undetected and unreported.

Some of the most egregious examples cited in the report were those of several female residents being sexually molested by a male attendant, and an incident where an aide walked into a female resident's room, shouted, "I'm tired of your ass," hit the resident in the face and broke her nose.

There are innumerable instances of verbal abuse; attendants calling the residents "bitch," "stupid," and "blob," just to name a few.

Another incident cited in the government report which, in my view, is even more intolerable and unforgivable, was when a discussion took place between a state inspector and the home's Director of Nursing. When the inspector asked about a female resident who appeared to have been sexually abused, the director replied, "Maybe she fell on a broomstick."

Many of us have heard personal horror stories of neglect, abuse, and theft directly from relatives of those confined in nursing homes. That shocking, scandalous, and disgraceful treatment apparently is widespread, and should not be allowed to continue!

In 1997 there were 17,000 nursing facilities in the United States, according to the National Center for Health Statistics (NCHS). Service was provided to 1.6 million residents, and 2.4 million residents were discharged or died the previous year.

More than 90% of those residing in nursing homes are sixty-five years of age or older, and almost half of those are eighty-five or older.

Some of the information from the NCHS is confusing about the daily charge for these facilities. It appears to be based on the level of care, the certification status, and the ownership. There is a wide range of prices listed; the lowest being $98 daily, to the highest of $217. There are homes operated by the government, proprietary homes, non-profit homes, and both Medicaid-certified and Medicare-certified homes. Certified nurse aides are responsible for the majority of care.

I refuse to accept that a nursing home will be the only option available to those who become incapacitated and unable to care for themselves in the future. There has to be a better way!

Nor do I accept the inevitability of helplessness and dependency in old age. I believe that it's possible to remain healthy and independent for a very long time, possibly until it is time for death; the heart will simply stop beating because the body can no longer sustain itself.

CHAPTER IV – Illness and Disease.

There are many more potentially serious problems for the elderly than the physical changes already discussed. Arthritis (the type known as osteoarthritis) is much too common in older people and sometimes disabling, or at least is a contributing factor in the decreased mobility of many.

Obviously older people are not as strong as they once were, reflexes are often not as quick, and there may be problems with balance and coordination.

Some vision problems can't be avoided as we age, but with proper treatment, many can be corrected. A relatively small percentage of the elderly are blind; only 1% in those over the age of sixty-five, and 3% in those over the age of eighty-five. But there is always the risk of very serious eye diseases such as Macular Degeneration, Glaucoma, and Cataracts.

Many older people will also suffer from hearing loss, particularly those who have worked in noisy, industrial environments, or those who listened to very loud music for many years. Of course there can be other causes of deafness. This can also seriously affect one's ability to communicate well with others, which may lead to isolation and solitude.

I've read that our sense of taste and sense of smell are diminished as we grow older. However, I have experienced no such thing; and others with whom I've spoken tell me they are not aware of any differences.

As we age, there may be some degree of short-term memory loss; perhaps we can't recall names and places as quickly as we once did. But there is no evidence to indicate there is severe mental decline, unless of course, there is some kind of disease.

On the website of the American Association of Neurological Surgeons, I recently learned that significant memory loss is not inevitable as we grow older, that the degree of loss cannot be directly linked to age.

That same source indicates there is solid scientific evidence to support the fact that eating certain foods can enhance brain functions, and that physical activity is closely linked to life-long brain health.

According to available statistics, there are approximately 4 million Americans who are currently afflicted with Alzheimer's Disease, and of course it is anticipated that the number will increase. But we shouldn't assume that, if we live long enough, we will be stricken with Alzheimer's.

In the past we have been given information by medical professionals that was not always correct. It is now known that many conditions which were thought to be age-related are not.

It is not a normal part of ageing to have dementia; to have osteoporosis; to be incontinent; to suffer from diverticulitis or colon problems; digestive problems and constipation; to be nervous or have anxiety attacks; to be depressed; to lack energy, or to be stolid and lethargic.

Until very recently, it was sometimes thought that elevated blood pressure levels in the elderly were normal, especially in individuals over the age of seventy-five. There was often a tendency by doctors to ignore the increased levels because of the misconception that "100 plus your age" was a normal systolic (top) pressure, and that has proven to be untrue.

All of us know that it is extremely important to keep blood

pressure under control to reduce the increased risk of strokes and heart attacks.

Strokes are the third greatest cause of death in older Americans, and high blood pressure, or hypertension, is the primary cause. They are also the number one cause of disability in the United States, with more than 3 million people currently living with brain damage.

It is crucial that more attention be given to all patients with the potential for disease. Early diagnosis and treatment can obviate the risk of long-term disability and/or death.

Even though they are not a "normal" part of ageing, many of the conditions, ailments, and diseases mentioned are quite common. Some can be prevented with early detection and intervention; others can be managed effectively.

For many years most of us indulged in activities and conduct that did not promote good physical and mental health.

But in all fairness, some of the damage we inflicted was because of our own ignorance; i.e., we knew nothing about the dangers of cigarette smoking for many years. And who knew that lying in the sun for hours without sunscreen protection could cause cancer!

A report in 1996 from the office of the U.S. Surgeon General alerted Americans to the reality that our sedentary lifestyles are killing us. The report reiterated the same depressing news we had heard before: that hypertension, diabetes, heart disease, and colon cancer can be directly related to a sedentary lifestyle.

We were told that even moderate amounts of exercise may help ease arthritis symptoms, improve our mood and mental acuity, relieve depression and/or anxiety. And certainly it can help in the prevention of obesity.

Unfortunately, there are some older citizens who have constructed invisible barriers that won't allow them to participate in certain activities because they think they're "too old." Many fear that they will fall and break a bone, or that the risk of incurring a serious injury is just too great. The notion that you are too old is nonsense, in my opinion.

Naturally if you are frail, have osteoporosis, problems with coordination and balance, common sense dictates that you shouldn't attempt anything that will place you in harm's way. But your doctor, or some other health professional, can advise you on "sit-down" and other appropriate exercises. Of course a physical examination may be warranted before undertaking any kind of strenuous activity or exercise regime.

As consumers, old and young alike, we must make every effort to educate ourselves on various health issues; enabling us to determine the best course of action for our own personal needs and goals. This is a responsibility which we cannot afford to ignore.

Inactivity, poor eating habits, and an attitude that taking a pill is the answer to everything, are serious issues and should require meaningful discussions between doctor and patient.

According to The Disaster Center of the CDC, the five leading causes of death for those in the U. S. who are sixty-five and over are: (1) Heart Disease (2) Cancers (3) Strokes (4) Chronic Obstructive Pulmonary Disease (COPD) and (5) Pneumonia and influenza. All accidents, including motor vehicle, are listed as the 7th leading cause of death.

The cost of health care is enormous. A report from the U.S. General Accounting Office (GAO) in 1995 estimated that the cost of medication-related problems in the elderly, i.e., improper dosing, over-dosing, and adverse reactions, amounted to approximately $20 billion a year in hospital stays. And as previously mentioned, an estimated $20.2 billion is spent every year on injuries that are related to falls.

It's also estimated that approximately $7 billion is spent annually on various medications used for heartburn and Gastroesophageal Reflux Disease (GERD). Of course that is not restricted to senior citizens.

And the U.S. Government predicts that Medicare recipients are projected to spend $1.8 trillion on prescription drugs over the next ten years. Those numbers are incomprehensible – they "boggle" the mind!

Drug companies profit greatly from older Americans. An organization for health care consumers has reported that in a six-month period in the year 2003, prices of the fifty most prescribed drugs for senior citizens rose, on average, almost three and one-half times the rate of inflation. These included some allergy drugs, estrogen replacement, beta blockers, cholesterol-lowering drugs, anti-osteoporotic drugs, drugs for arthritis treatment, and many others.

It is especially difficult for low-income seniors to pay for their prescription drugs. They sometimes must make a choice between their medication and other necessities of life.

The statistics, costs and numbers, are public information, and readily available to members of Congress and the departments who oversee the health and welfare of all Americans.

The research that is done, the investigations that are made, the numbers that are compiled, are all fine; but, it seems to me, that the *focus* should be on what action can be taken after that data is collected. What good are the reports if they continue to gather dust on someone's desk?

CHAPTER V – Attitude and Action.

Many of us did not learn over the years to be more involved in, and responsible for our own physical and mental well-being. And regardless of one's age, it is never too late to change, and improve the quality of life. Never accept the words, "you're too old for that" from yourself or from anyone else. That is just so very wrong.

There are a number of reasons that partially explain why many have neglected themselves; for much of their adult lives they were taking care of their families. They were giving, loving, generous and selfless when it came to caring for others, and had little or no time for themselves. Taking time out for relaxation, fun and entertainment, exercise, or just a little pampering, would be unthinkable. And as we all know, old habits are not always easy to break, but because of a new attitude many are able to conquer them.

More needs to be said about the *stigma* confronting us as we glide, slide, or creep into old age, and that is that senior citizens themselves are partially responsible for perpetuating that stigma. Of course it is not done deliberately, and such a remark may be a personal affront to some.

I think there are a significant number who actually accept the idea that as we age we become unproductive and useless, with no longer a purpose in life. It is the belief of some that they will be weak and feeble, stricken with serious illness or disease, unable to care for themselves.

There are those who live in fear of leaving their house; too much of a risk. They isolate themselves, and have little or no social interaction. They spend a lot of time watching their television sets, and not much of anything else. And they are convinced that it is just a matter of time until they lose their independence.

There is often too much time spent dwelling on the past; what they were, what they did, and living with a palpable sense of sadness and regret. They believe that the future is marred by gloom and doom.

It is my opinion that a much more positive way to avoid depression, memory decline, and those other maladies for which they're preparing themselves, would be to find constructive things to do – challenging and interesting projects – that are physically and mentally stimulating.

I see no advantages to a fatalistic outlook; it limits your power to overcome negativity and pursue a positive course which will guarantee that you, and you alone, are in control of your own destiny. A brighter attitude, mood, and temperament will be the undeniable result, and your long-held belief of what one becomes in old age will not be a self-fulfilling prophecy.

A few years ago I was surprised by a visit from an old friend I hadn't seen in almost 25 years. It didn't take me long to see that she had actually become the "stereotypical" old person (at the time she was fifty-nine or sixty). Physically she looked fine, but after being around her for only a brief period, I determined that she really *was not* fine. She habitually complained of minor aches and pains; a toothache, a headache, a stiff neck, or a sore foot.

She had little or no interest in going out and doing some fun things. At my insistence, she agreed to a few "outings," and constantly complained about one thing or another; she was too tired, the sun was too bright, she didn't want to walk anymore, etc.

At some point I asked her if she had brought a camera, that it would be nice to get a few pictures. She quickly informed me that, no, she had not brought a camera, that she was too old to be taking pictures. There were some other comments made with reference to ageing and the concomitant consequences.

Not only did she appear to be miserable during the entire visit, she also made me miserable. No one enjoys the company of a person who is disagreeable and moody.

She was entirely different from the friend of years ago. It was surely more than the ageing process that caused the change in personality and attitude. My theory is that she experienced some kind of trauma; some mental, physical, or spiritual incident that had a devastating effect.

I won't accept the idea that an individual can change so dramatically only because she is confronted with old age.

I think the "irascible old man," or the "cranky old lady," were irascible and cranky their entire lives. Those are often the people whose conduct becomes even worse in old age because they think they now have a "license" to behave badly. They believe others will overlook what they do, or make excuses for their actions. Their unpleasantness and ill humor are heightened as they age. If they were contentious and argumentative before, now it is exaggerated.

We know there are eccentrics at every age; we also know that there are older people who are not pleasant to be around. Some are bitter and angry, but I believe that is a relatively small number, and does not represent the majority of America's senior citizens.

Some criticisms of older people are probably justified. For example, if you think, "that old man smells bad," you're probably right. Sadly, many older people do smell bad; they wear the same clothes for days without washing them. They seem to think if there are no dirt or food stains on the clothes that it's okay to wear them indefinitely.

And a few appear to have an aversion to bathing. As a concession to the sensibilities of all, I won't expound my views on indifference to personal hygiene; and concede that it's not possible for everyone to bathe daily. If incapacitated, it's difficult to consider a bath or shower as a top priority. But if dry skin is a concern, there are many effective remedies, none of which require you to stop bathing.

Another frequent complaint against old people is that they have bad breath. Of course wearing dentures can contribute to this, and good dental care is important. However, there can be many causes for halitosis, which a physician may determine.

The above criticism might apply to any age group; bad breath and body odor are not the exclusive domain of senior citizens, and let it not be said that *malodorous* is synonymous with *old age*.

Actually I did recently learn that sometime there is a pronounced odor in those who are older that is not present in younger people, and that there is a logical explanation for it. That gives us even more reason to pay sedulous attention to our personal hygiene.

An interesting discovery was apparently made through Japanese research. The company, Shiseido Beautech Co., Ltd., has found that Nonenal, which is a substance found in body odor, increases with ageing. It is a type of unsaturated aldehyde and has an unpleasant and greasy odor, with a grassy nuance, according to the research. It is rarely found in the body odor of people in their 20s and 30s, but is found in the body odor of women and men in their 40s and older.

More scientific details are given for the increase in Nonenal, but Shiseido explains that basically after analyzing sebum, which is secreted by glands in the skin, and is much more prevalent in the elderly, that it has a large amount of lipid peroxide. Therefore, it is prone to oxidative degradation. So, the sebum is more likely to cause the formation of Nonenal, and that sometimes causes the unpleasant odor. (That's probably more than you wanted to know).

Still another common criticism, especially from children, is "I don't want to talk to him/her; he keeps telling me to speak up, to stop mumbling; he can't hear a thing I say." Often, because of hearing loss, he or she has a legitimate reason for asking people to repeat themselves. But many, I feel, are selective in what they do and do not hear. They often are just miserable, and wish to inflict misery and despair on those around them. Frequently they become impatient and agitated, particularly with lively and energetic children.

But that does not reflect the disposition of most seniors, and the consensus should not be that such behavior is characteristic, or typical.

Recently the controversial subject of senior citizens' driving habits was a topic of interest at a social event I attended. And some of the questions pertaining to the issuance of drivers' license were discussed; age limits, annual driving tests, and refresher driving courses.

The majority agreed that after age 70, every driver should be required to take a driving test each year before a license can be renewed. Most were also in favor of mandatory refresher driving courses, but no one could agree on how frequently those should take place.

Many of the participants in these discussions were people over the age of fifty; some were considerably older. A few believed that mandating a different set of rules for the elderly would be an unmistakable form of discrimination.

I don't think it is discrimination, and would willingly agree to be tested at my present age. It is probably not necessary, but admittedly there are some people in their sixties who have diminished cognitive skills, slower reflexes and reaction time, as well as impaired vision; some see well in daylight hours, but poorly at night.

And actually taking a driving test with a well-trained instructor observing, would be invaluable in determining if you are still capable of driving a motor vehicle. It is always easier for someone else to see our mistakes, and point out areas in which we need improvement.

I think compulsory driving courses could also benefit the driver, increasing awareness of their own capabilities, or potential deficiencies. Whatever measures can be taken to assist in accident prevention should be seriously considered.

According to the AAA Foundation for Traffic Safety, a person over age sixty-five is almost twice as likely as a middle-aged driver to die in a car crash. Those over seventy-five years of age are two and one-half times as likely, and those over age eighty-five are 3.72 times as likely to die in a crash as those drivers who are between the age of fifty-five and sixty-four.

Older drivers are sometimes responsible for accidents in which their vehicle is not actually involved. They may make an improper lane change, an unlawful turn, or some other ill-timed traffic maneuver; another driver, acting defensively is then unable to avoid a collision with someone else. The older driver is completely oblivious, and continues on his merry way.

In our driving habits, and other areas of our lives, there is room for improvement. With awareness, and a favorable inclination to accept change and make a few concessions, we can dispel some long-held myths and misconceptions.

CHAPTER VI – Positive Aspects of Ageing.

Senior citizens are not a monolithic and homogeneous group; we're all different, and should be accepted for our individuality. We have different abilities, interests, and gifts; an accumulation of knowledge, wisdom, talent, and experience that is invaluable.

Many are remaining very active; contributing much, doing great things for their communities. They're changing the stereotypical definition, and refuse to be labeled as senile, helpless, dependent, and just "taking up space."

Someone told me the story of a woman in her seventies who was truly inspirational. She apparently realized how intolerable her personal situation had become when she was unable to lift a large bag after making purchases at a grocery store. This was not acceptable, and after returning home, she immediately set about making changes in her life. She refused to accept the notion that once you reach a certain age you must "give up," and since you're "over the hill" the rest must all be "downhill." She believed that she could become stronger and healthier.

Since there was a need for professional assistance in the areas of nutrition and exercise, she consulted the experts. After some advice, and a few suggestions from a nutritionist and an exercise guru, or personal trainer, she was well on her way. She began doing strength-training and cardiovascular exercises, changed her eating habits, and made other lifestyle adjustments. The time, energy, and effort expended apparently resulted in a happier, healthier, and much more physically fit individual.

That is a great example of what one can accomplish, regardless of age. Of course determination, dedication, desire, and *discipline*, are necessary in any worthwhile endeavor.

I personally can attest to the benefits derived from eating properly, exercising, maintaining a positive attitude, and rarely walking away from a challenge.

I know a sixty-five-year-old woman who can bench press 100 pounds, and do twenty-five consecutive push-ups. She walks two to three miles a day, five days a week, and is much more agile, with more stamina than many thirty- to forty-year-old people I know.

Perhaps you have absolutely no desire to do push-ups, and couldn't care less about bench pressing anything. And that's fine, too.

Walking is an exercise that almost everyone can do that is actually fun, and can be even more so if you find friends or family members who will walk with you. It doesn't even have to feel as if you're exercising. It's great!

Following a back injury many years ago, I began brisk walking on a regular basis at the suggestion of my doctor. I have continued this daily routine for more than twenty years. I believe it has had a huge impact on my physical abilities. Without this, and other specific exercises designed for the care of my back, I would at least be a semi-invalid, possibly requiring some form of walking aid; a walker or cane.

There are many examples of how the "very old" who are still healthy and energetic, continue to lead productive lives. They are involved in politics, charities, and volunteer work in their communities. Many are still a part of the regular work force. *Seniors USA*, an online magazine, has listed a few of the more impressive ones:

A one hundred-year-old man, who edits a medical journal at a hospital, arrives at work at 8 A.M. daily.

A ninety-two-year-old man works forty hours a week as an efficiency expert at a plant that makes steel strings for guitars and banjos.

A ninety-three-year-old woman who has worked in the same real estate office for fifty years can still type 120 words per minute.

A ninety-five-year-old man still cuts hair at the barbershop he opened in 1925.

And most of us have heard or read about the Delany sisters; Dr. Annie Elizabeth Delany, and Sarah Delany, affectionately known as Bessie and Sadie. One was a school teacher and one was a dentist, the second black woman licensed to practice dentistry in the state of New York. Bessie died in 1995 at the age of one hundred four years; Sadie died in 1999 at age one hundred nine.

In 1992 the sisters published a book called *Having Our Say; The Delany Sisters' First 100 Years.* The book was very successful, and even became a Broadway play.

In 1994 they published a second book: *The Delany Sisters Book of Everyday Wisdom.* After the death of her sister, Sadie wrote still another book called *On My Own At 107; Reflections On Life Without Bessie.*

According to information from the U.S. Department of Health and Human Services in 2003, there was no accurate count of centenarians, but it was estimated at more than 60,000; many remaining independent and relatively healthy until death.

The *Seniors USA* online magazine points out that many people in the present work force are planning to work past the age of sixty-five. The Bureau of Labor Statistics corroborates that, and says the number of older workers is steadily increasing. Even though many companies do discriminate, there are some who value the older worker.

There are those who must continue to work for financial reasons, but countless numbers work simply because they enjoy it, and see no reason to stop as long as they remain healthy, and can be productive. The idea of retirement simply doesn't appeal to everyone.

The baby-boomers who are fast becoming seniors are doing a lot to squash many of the prevailing myths and stereotypes. Those healthy, energetic, and active people will continue to disprove popular-held notions, which, in turn, will help to change much of society's negative attitude.

The "boomers" probably see ageing as another phase, another passage in their life; perhaps a time to explore new horizons, a time for traveling and pursuing adventures about which they've only dreamed.

I don't believe it is uncharitable or self-centered to take time now to think about yourself, to consider your own needs and desires. Concentrating on a path to improve your life, on ways to look and feel better, and be happier, will enable you to reach out to others, and exemplify all that is positive and affirmative, while growing old gracefully. Remember the truism, "you can't love others unless you first love yourself." And can you really love yourself if you're tentative, doubtful, and uncertain about the future? And there definitely *is* a future!

CHAPTER VII – Conclusion.

It is necessary that interest in, and concern for, our physical and mental health begin early in life. This should be just as important, if not more so, as planning for our financial future. One only has to become seriously ill to realize that the need for good health surpasses the need for all other things we believe to be so essential in our lives. We then quickly become cognizant of our misplaced priorities.

It is our responsibility and duty to take care of ourselves, and not continuously abuse our body and our mind. And I'm not so old that I've forgotten most of us are not willing to give up some of the "bad" habits considered to be not only fun, but also are a part of our passage into serious adult maturity.

But we only need to look around us, and to read the medical information with which we are inundated, to know that even children and adolescents are indulging in lifestyles that are potentially deadly.

We're told by the health professionals that obesity among adults, as well as children, has become an epidemic in the United States. There are many children who have high blood pressure, high cholesterol, diabetes, and myriad illnesses that were once considered to be restricted to adults.

The National Institutes of Health (NIH) reported in the year 2000 that nearly two-thirds of adults in the U.S. were overweight or obese. And the prevalence is steadily increasing.

In that same year there were approximately 300,000 premature adult deaths that were directly attributable to unhealthy dietary habits and lack of physical activity.

Recent statistics from both national and international health organizations indicate that Americans are among the fattest people on earth.

That information is disturbing, and it seems that only recently have these issues begun to resonate among parents, teachers, health-care professionals, and those in a position to initiate change.

It is unacceptable to see so many children and adolescents lead a sedentary life, with little or no physical activity, and indulge in poor eating habits.

But I believe it's even more indefensible for adults to engage in that kind of destructive behavior, and lack of discipline. They should try to be a positive role model for the young.

Of course the problems didn't occur overnight; the health professionals have been telling us for a long time that our lifestyles were detrimental to our health, but no one seemed anxious to do anything about it. Now it's time!

Some health professionals believe about 75% of illness and disease is a direct result of our lifestyles. I tend to think the percentage may be even greater.

I accept without question that there are outside forces, over which we have little or no control, that can have a damaging effect on our health and our lives. There are often toxins in the air we breathe. Harmful substances such as asbestos and lead have been found in schools and the workplace, mercury is in the fish we eat, our water is sometimes contaminated, and because of heredity, many people are predisposed to certain illnesses and disease.

But don't give up! If you can physically move your limbs, and if you can think rationally, I believe it is possible to improve your quality of life. And I contend that *quality* is far more important than *quantity.*

We should not expect miracles from physicians or depend so completely on pills as a panacea. Our common sense and good judgment tell us we should avoid things that are harmful. And it's crucial that we avail ourselves of all the information, counseling, advice, and services we can find, to assist us in making rational, reasonable decisions regarding our health and every facet of our lives.

I am often reminded that America is a wonderful country. We have so much, and are blessed in many, many ways. But we aren't perfect; and for all that is good, I believe a very real need exists for better care, more respect, appreciation, and recognition of our senior citizens.

There are cultures who revere their elders; Japan immediately comes to mind. And from my own observations and discussions with others, Hispanics also appear to be very "family-oriented," and do all that's within their power to avoid placing an ill or disabled relative in a nursing home. They are cared for in their own home. To do anything less appears to be unacceptable; "discarding" a family member is obviously not a part of their culture.

There are probably other societies in which the elderly are honored and venerated. It is my fervent hope that one day America will proudly honor their own, and hold them in high esteem.

Older people have acquired skills and wisdom they did not possess in their youth. I am thankful for those skills and that wisdom; and if I am to be judged by others, then it should be for my character, my actions, my attitude, my attributes, and my contributions.

We senior citizens must forget the suggestion that we are "too old" to participate in, and contribute to the community in which we live, and society as a whole.

We must ignore the popular belief of some that getting old means being sick, frail, and helpless; we cannot allow society to reduce us to a useless, ineffective, inferior relic.

We must remain optimistic and positive, with enthusiasm and a zest for living; and believe with the essence of our being that if we've reached old age as a healthy, vigorous, strong, self-assured, and happy individual, that there is absolutely no reason to think we can't continue for a very long time.

With the expectation that by the year 2030 one of every five Americans will be sixty-five years old or older, there will probably be a financial impact on society, particularly in our health care system.

But there are solutions, one of which is to have healthier citizens. We know how to do that – with careful planning and preparation, and the practical application of what we've learned.

It's essential that preventive and rehabilitative medicine become a viable part of our health care system, with attention given to everyone, long before they're old.

Effective alternatives to our present-day nursing homes are badly needed. An affordable insurance plan that will cover the cost of long-term and comprehensive care in an individual's home should be made available to everyone.

The care received should be based on the patient's needs, and not on their financial status. Equal treatment for all must be demanded.

In my view, there is a lot that can, and should, be done. And I feel that only when the plight of the elderly, especially those residing in nursing homes, is fully recognized, and generates sufficient interest for commitment and change, will there be satisfactory solutions. I am optimistic that these goals are attainable, and one day will reach fruition.

Printed in the United States
23909LVS00004B/255